D0717363

Rediscover the power of creativity,
curiosity and imagination

THE LITTLE BOOK OF

WONDER

BERNADETTE RUSSELL

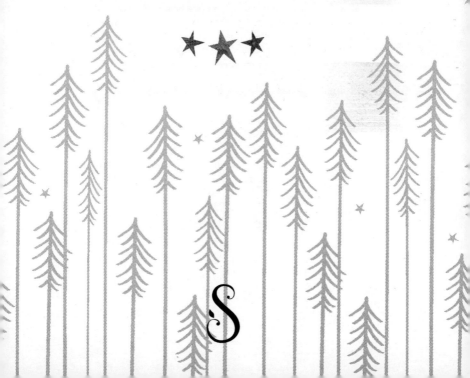

★ ★ ★

S

First published in Great Britain in 2018 by Orion Spring
an imprint of The Orion Publishing Group Ltd
Carmelite House, 50 Victoria Embankment
London EC4Y 0DZ

An Hachette UK Company

1 3 5 7 9 10 8 6 4 2

A CIP catalogue record for this book is available from the British Library.

ISBN: 978 1 4091 8301 3
ISBN (Ebook): 978 1 4091 8302 0

Printed in Great Britain by CPI Group (UK) Ltd, Croydon, CR0 4YY

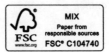

MIX
Paper from
responsible sources
FSC® C104740

www.orionbooks.co.uk

ORION
SPRING

CONTENTS

Introduction   5

1. The Wonder of You   13
2. Into the Woods   32
3. Curiouser and Curiouser   46
4. Practical Magic   60
5. We Are All Artists   77
6. The Road Less Travelled   93
7. Positive Thinking   105

Further reading   122
Acknowledgements   123
About the author   126

INTRODUCTION

★ ★ ★

We are the music makers,
And we are the dreamers of dreams,
Wandering by lone sea-breakers,
And sitting by desolate streams;—
World-losers and world-forsakers,
On whom the pale moon gleams:
Yet we are the movers and shakers
Of the world for ever, it seems.

FROM *ODE* BY ARTHUR O'SHAUGHNESSY

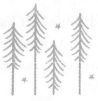

We are surrounded by wonders. Yet it is so easy for us to become weighed down with chores, worries and work, to become so preoccupied and inward-looking that we begin to forget that we live in an incredible world, full of beauty, that we and our fellow humans are amazing too, capable of great and surprising things. For the most part children are much better at experiencing wonder at the world and themselves. This is an invitation to revisit the wonderland of your childhood (or to invent one for yourself if your childhood wasn't so wonderful).

This book contains simple, creative and fun exercises, to encourage you to use your curiosity and imagination. They will lift you out of the ordinary and allow you to be in awe of the world again, the way you are when you've fallen in love, been inspired by art or nature, after a wild night out, or on a special occasion like a wedding, an eclipse, or the birth of a child.

I'd also like to invite you to do the important things your heart craves but which you put aside for more grown-up matters: that novel you've always wanted to write, the old friend you would love to get back in touch with, the camping trip you never make time for, the carpentry course you consider but never get round to. The things that help you experience wonder.

Exploring these things will bring you so much pleasure and inspiration. Here are a few instructions to start you off on your journey: Look up. Listen. Daydream. Seek out magic. Pursue learning all your life. Never stop asking questions. Enjoy not knowing sometimes. Be still. Keep moving. Allow yourself to be an artist, scientist, creator, inventor, and explorer. Embrace the wonder of being alive right here, right now on this incredible planet, with these, your fellow travellers.

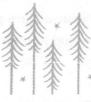

*M*ost scientific research into wonder concludes that experiencing it makes us aware that we are part of something bigger than ourselves, such as a community, humanity in general, or the whole universe. This encourages helpful 'pro-social' behaviours – we might perhaps become more interested in helping others, giving to charity or volunteering. These behaviours have proven health benefits: for example charitable giving is known to reduce stress and increase a general feeling of wellbeing, and being connected to a community promotes longevity and increases our overall happiness.

It's a wonderful world

When we become aware of how amazing the world is, we are more likely to want to look after it. Recent publicity about the incredible biodiversity of our oceans and the threats posed by plastic pollution has led to much greater public awareness and this in turn has led to a change in attitudes – there has already been a 30 per cent drop in plastic bags on the seabed. By being in awe of the natural world we become more aware of how precious and vital it is, and more active in helping to protect our environment by changing our behaviour.

Humans are awesome

Considering the incredible past achievements and future potential of human beings allows us to feel hopeful and optimistic about the future. Focusing on the things humans have got right, the advancements we have made, and the obstacles we have overcome gives us pleasure in experiencing the wonder of human beings. This has a positive effect on our mental health.

My story

I was working as an actor at the Edinburgh Festival, performing in three different shows, which required me to run all over town, quickly put on that show's costume, get myself on stage, and remember the lines without mixing the shows up. It was massive fun, fuelled by reckless amounts of coffee and pre-show adrenaline. At the end of each day, which was usually sometime in the early hours of the next morning, weary, footsore and anxious, I lay awake with glittering eyes, worrying that if I didn't sleep I wouldn't have enough energy left for tomorrow. I was exhausted. The corner of my eye felt like it was being tugged by miniature pixies.

Sometimes I didn't worry though. I became distracted by the witchy beauty of the shadows of the tree branches on the ceiling, and I listened to the wind rattling empty cans of something or other outside. Spooky, desolate, a melancholy city soundscape. I told my friend about the shadows and the wind, and he said, 'I found this' and showed me *The Book of Scottish Ghost Stories*. He said, 'Let's read some.'

And so we did.

We sat up, read each other ghost stories, and rediscovered the wonder of listening, being read to and reading aloud. And perhaps because all words are magic words, I did sleep better that night. After that, every night, after the shows came down, after watching late-night comedians in sticky-floored pub basements, after last orders of peaty whiskies, and chips eaten with scalded fingers out of paper cones, we came home and read aloud to each other. It was magical.

When I got back to London, I asked my friend Gill if we could organise a storytelling night in her café, and that's what we did. The very first time there were just a few of us, plus a plate of samosas, a bottle of wine and some home-made cakes. Over the course of the next ten years, we continued to hold our storytelling parties every month in London (and later in Brighton too), and they became legendary. We were accompanied by a raggle-taggle group of wonderful people: several magicians, a small orchestra, a hula hoop champion, a burlesque dancer, a cosmologist, a self-proclaimed witch, a philosopher, an anaesthetist, a group of octogenarian knitters from Essex, some Morris dancers and a ukulele-playing poet to name a few. We played musical chairs and pass the parcel. We encouraged each other and our visitors to listen, to play, and to immerse themselves in a world of imagination. We told, and listened to, and wrote, and worked with hundreds of stories and writers. We baked hundreds of cakes. Our audience wrote wishes in the winter sky with sparklers and posted miniature stories they had written at our events through complete strangers' letterboxes. We encouraged mischief. When we ran out of words we made new ones up.

What we discovered in that time was this huge appetite in people for the things which we are usually encouraged to abandon when childhood is over, once we get busy earning money, accumulating stuff and worries. Things that involve using your imagination for its own sake, listening, joining in, daring to be silly and brave and eccentric. We created an inclusive space where everyone felt at home, where anything felt possible. We did this from nothing, because we wanted to and so we went ahead and did it. You can do this too.

During the last year I have met with and chatted to scientists, philosophers, magicians and artists among others, about the meaning and importance of wonder, and how their work and lives are impacted by it. You will read about them later, and there is information about each of them in the back of the book.

As for me, I don't have any special qualifications that have emboldened me to wrote about wonder, except a restless curiosity and a hunger for getting as much as I can out of life while I'm here.

That's all you need, so come with me to wonderland, and allow yourself to dream ...

Bernadette Russell

CHAPTER 1

THE WONDER OF YOU

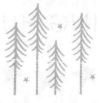

*C*ongratulations, you are part of an incredible species that has achieved and is capable of astonishing things. You too are capable of astonishing things. Human creativity is endless. Art, scientific discoveries and inventions are a source of wonder and inspiration for us all.

Your mission:

To give yourself permission and time to play, dream and investigate the incredible wonder of you as an individual, with all your attributes, talents and achievements. To also explore and celebrate the wonder of being human, considering and learning about all we have done in the past, and all we have the potential to do in the future. To have fun and get creative while doing so!

AMAZING HUMANS

We have been pretty busy over the years: bashing rocks into useful-shaped tools, building space rockets and dreaming up the internet. Here are some of my favourite human inventions:

Fire

It seems likely that we managed fire control around 300,000 years ago, and from then on, it was easier for us to keep warm, fend off predators and cook. I like to imagine that this was when all the fun started, like parties and night-time sing-alongs. Our ancestors experimented, persevered and probably perished getting this basic thing going. As a regular camper, I appreciate this very much.

Shoes

Protecting our feet from rocks, nettles, and things that bite, there's evidence of shoes dating back 40,000 years. After that, it became possible to explore and travel much more safely. I'm very grateful I live in a world where I don't have to fashion my own footwear out of oak leaves.

Penicillin

A turning point in human history was when Dr Fleming discovered a tool to cure diseases completely, all from a mouldy Petri dish, which just goes to show washing up isn't *always* a good thing.

Of course there are loads more inventions I admire: the wheel, the printing press, chocolate biscuits, but now …

It's your turn! Consider which three human inventions/discoveries inspire you. Find out when and how that happened (they're *always* more awe-inspiring the more you find out).

My top three inventions/discoveries and how they came about:

1. _____

2. _____

3. _____

I hope you feel inspired by what humans have achieved. You are part of the species that did these incredible things!

Next, let's consider art …

HUMAN CREATIVITY

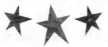

We have carved our likenesses into mountains, launched music into space, inspired peace (and begun wars) with words. Art is a way of expressing what it is to be alive; it helps remind us of the incredible possibilities of being human. It is inspirational to enjoy creativity for its own sake, and to remind ourselves of the effort and work involved in its making.

<u>Over to you!</u> Think about the art you like: a child's drawing, a busker playing on your way into work, a favourite TV show. Revisit a few of your favourite things and let yourself enjoy them again. Answer these questions for each thing you love ...

I love ... _____

How I first discovered it ... _____

I love it because ... _____

It makes me feel ... _____

<u>Spread the wonder</u>: find someone who might be inspired too – and introduce them to it.

<u>My dreamtime</u>: now ask yourself what *you* would like to create if anything were possible. If thoughts like 'but I can't' pop up, acknowledge them, and put them to one side. Just let yourself dream. Make yourself a promise to try at least one of them in the next twelve months.

Write your dreams here:

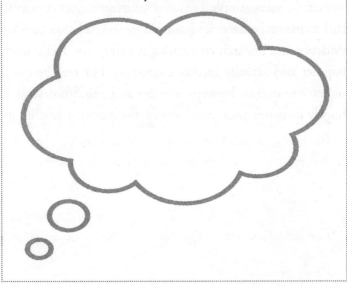

Now you've been reminded of how amazing other humans can be, let's focus on you.

BEING IN THE MOMENT

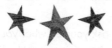

Watching my dog Lola joyfully tearing around the park is my daily reminder of the joy of being present in the moment. I've suffered from anxiety most of my life, and can confirm that daily practice of mindfulness helps enormously. Mindfulness is simply bringing your attention gently to this moment in time, without judgement. There's tons of evidence and research confirming it makes you feel calmer, happier and actually increases curiosity. For me there is a direct connection between wonder and mindfulness as it hugely increases your awareness of the moment you are in.

Your body knows exactly what to do. Let's stay focused on your amazing body for a while ...

BODY TALK

I chatted with Dr Bentley Crudgington (a medical education researcher at Manchester University) about the wonder of our bodies and he said: 'When you see a lamb leaping about, there is a perfect example of a creature enjoying how incredible it is to have a body – just utter joy, excitement, and wonder. We need to remind ourselves to do that too.'

We all take our incredible bodies for granted, even the most health conscious among us. Just consider for a moment this amazing fact: human thigh bones are stronger than steel and four times stronger than concrete.

<u>Over to you!</u> Get curious about how you work. Go for taste buds if you're a foodie, eyes if you love photography, ears if you love music etc. Choose something about yourself you are intrigued by and investigate – then record your own amazing facts here (repeat as often as you like):

The amazing thing about _____ *is* _____

See? You're incredible.

EVERY BODY

Exercise can remind you that your body can be strong, tough, enduring and can bring you fun and happiness. You might be amazed by what you achieve.

Find something you love. It could be strenuous, like army fitness training through lakes of mud, or simply walking in the woods, swimming in your local lido, or learning to tango.

It can do so much good, including: reduce your risk of heart disease, stroke, and cancer by up to 50 per cent, boost self-esteem, sleep quality and energy, plus reduce stress and depression!

Dr Crudgington said: 'Imagine how much joy there'd be if all the people who said I could never dance, I have no rhythm, just went and danced in their own rhythm. Then perhaps they would realise it doesn't matter.'

I hope you find trying out new exercises inspiring, whatever your level of fitness, as it is new experiences that most inspire wonder!

THE STORY OF YOU

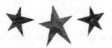

We've established that our bodies are amazing, and that being present is hugely beneficial. Now I'd like to focus on the wonder-full story of your life so far, then look to the future! It's good to pause sometimes and appreciate what you have experienced.

> <u>Try this</u>: write/draw/tell the story of your life. Focus on the positive and entertaining – it might have dramas, comedy, romance, and adventure. Include achievements, laughter, fun, and excitement. Choose someone you trust who's a sympathetic listener and tell them your story. Enjoy telling the wonderful story of your life. Let them ask questions.

See? Wasn't that a great story? However, if doing it made you consider things you'd like to have done … it's not too late. My friend Joy became an actor in her eighties – after a lifetime of working in an office, she just decided to give it a crack. Let's imagine what might come next for you …

Life can be wonderful, rich, and varied, if you allow it to be, and allow yourself to imagine it could be.

Once you know what you'd like, you can begin to explore what you need to do to make that possible.

Just in case you are thinking, it's all very well me wanting to do something but … let's move on to the superhero version of you.

SUPERHERO YOU

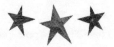

We all have something we are amazing at, or have the potential to be amazing at.

> <u>Try this</u>: Pair up with a friend and help each other devise a superhero name – as a silly example: 'Hedgewoman', if you're really good at gardening. You could even draw a picture of your superhero outfit.
>
> We all have something extraordinary about us – use this exercise to find out what it is about you.
>
> *My superpower is …*
>
> _____
>
> _____
>
> *My superhero name would be …*
>
> _____
>
> _____

Here is the drawing of superhero me ...

This is the 'wonder' version of you. It's a counter to the negative and self-critical thoughts that can pop up into your head as you go about your day.

But – you are a superhero of course, so these negative thoughts are no match for you. Make a habit of turning them into kinder thoughts and positive actions.

Here's an example

Thought: I'm not very good at my job and everyone at work thinks so too.

Could be: I'm going to focus on what I am good at and appreciate those things.

Action: I will work out what I need help with and who to ask.

Next time you identify a negative thought, try turning it around in the same way:

Thought: _____

Could be: _____

Action: _____

I AM AWESOME

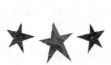

If you are being plagued by self-doubt, don't punish yourself — it happens to all of us. Lift yourself up by remembering you are awesome. Be specific.

<u>Hello, wonderful</u>: Sit down opposite a mirror. Then tell yourself all the things that make you wonderful, including your appearance, personality, achievements, attributes, talents etc. Feel free to continue for as long as you like.

<u>Pair up</u>: do this exercise with a friend. Each of you focuses on the things about the other that are rare, exceptional, surprising. Tell each other. We don't do this nearly enough. (Just warning you: there may be tears!) This brings us nicely on to love …

LOVE IS WONDERFUL

Kate Baily is a life coach who studied the Science of Happiness at Berkeley University. She reminded me that if we are ever in doubt of ourselves it is good to remember: we are all loved by someone, and we all love someone. This exercise is inspired by her.

<u>Try this</u>: inside this heart, write all the names of those whom you love.

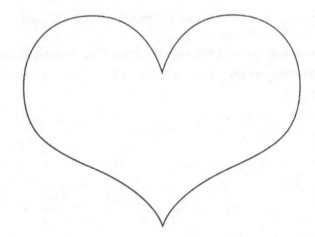

Then in this heart, write the names of everyone who loves you (pets included).

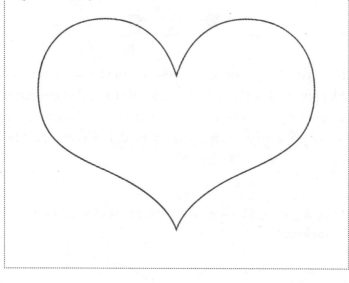

You see, you are loved, and you love. This in itself is cause for wonderment.

CHAPTER 2

INTO THE WOODS

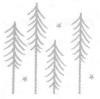

I was on my way home after a tiring couple of days working away. On the train I could hear the tinny bleating of music from headphones; everyone was looking down at their phones. Mine was flat, so I stared out of the window instead. It was a dull, grey November day, the sky heavy with clouds, mile after mile of flat damp fields dotted with cows chewing the cud.

Later, when I woke, the train had stopped between stations. I looked out of the window again. The huge sky above the flat expanse of sodden fields had turned crimson. Starlings swooped and soared, thousands of birds weaving a double helix against the clouds. Inside the carriage people looked up; some filmed the view on their phones, but after a while we all sat and watched. The quiet settled over us, a blanket of awe.

If someone set out to write a bucket list of places to go/things to do and see, it's doubtful if a mid-winter train journey between Leicester and London St Pancras on a damp Wednesday afternoon would make the list. But it was so beautiful.

I don't think there's any such thing as an ordinary day. If you pay attention and are present, there's much more chance of experiencing those moments of incredible beauty. Wonder is everywhere. You don't have to travel halfway around the world to be awestruck. You can just look around at home.

Your mission:

To slow down and appreciate the wonders of the natural world, focusing on the places closest to where you live. To enjoy the benefits to your mental and physical health by doing so. To help protect and cherish the natural world more as a result of your greater connection and understanding.

What is this life if, full of care,
We have no time to stand and stare.

FROM *LEISURE* BY W.H. DAVIES

WONDERLANDS

I visited the Natural History Museum in London and met with Lucy Minshall-Pearson, who works there as a science communicator. Lucy very kindly gave me a guided tour of the museum, and as we strolled around and chatted about the wonders of the natural world, Lucy said: 'All you have to do is go into your garden or the local park and lift up a log and look at all the creatures revealed underneath. The log used to be a living tree but is now home to beetles, that are food for birds, which are in turn food for other animals. You don't need to go anywhere special to experience how connected every living thing is.'

With this in mind, I'd like to invite you first of all to discover the natural wonders in your own little patch of earth, to explore them, learn about them, and use them to sustain and inspire you.

<u>My seven wonders</u>: It's easy for us to take our own surroundings for granted – this exercise is designed to make you appreciate your bit of the world!

Compile two lists of seven natural 'wonders' near your home, such as parks, nature reserves, woods, hills, mountains, or canals. One list is of places you already know and love (but maybe don't visit enough), the second a list of places you know of but haven't got round to going to yet. You may find that you have to do some investigating if you can't fill the list – go for it!

Start your lists here:

Places I love	Places I want to visit

Now draw your own personal 'Map of Wonders'. Your home should be on it, and as many places of natural beauty as you'd like to include. As you discover more you may add to it, keeping a written and visual record of your explorations. It could include drawings of trees, plants, animals that are there etc …

Now, switch off your phone and be an intrepid explorer — it's as simple as that! As you walk around, notice the sounds, sights, smells and physical sensations that are specific to this place. If your mind wanders off, bring it gently back to noticing the details of your environment.

If you like, you could make notes on your 'Map of Wonders' to keep a record of what you observed. If you're able, treat yourself to visiting one of these places at least once a week.

IN THE TREES

Nature provides us with many opportunities to slow down. Witnessing the gentleness, playfulness and tranquillity of nature can soothe us, taking us away from the hyperactivity of our day-to-day lives. Nature doesn't ask us to improve ourselves or produce results — we can just be. The Wildlife Trusts run a '30 Days Wild' campaign, during which participants try out wildlife activities every day for a month. Research conducted during this campaign confirmed an increase in participants' health and happiness. It also showed that the more people care for their environment and value the positive impact it has on their own lives, the more they want to protect it. It's a win-win.

Even though I live in central London, I visit the woods nearby every day to escape the hustle and bustle. I look out for squirrels scampering, birds swooping and playing in the sky, and different kinds of insects on the trees and water, and all my stresses melt away.

Try this: this is a Japanese practice called *shinrin-yoku*, or forest bathing. Walk slowly in the forest or woods, allowing yourself to wander without purpose, taking your time. Pay gentle attention to what you see, hear, taste, smell and feel. Notice the light filtering through the canopy of the trees, the different shades of green, birds singing, wind rustling the leaves, the sound and sight of creatures scampering about. Take deep breaths and enjoy the fresh air, reach out and touch the bark of a tree or the velvety softness of a leaf. Lie or sit down and just let yourself be.

Numerous scientific studies conducted by Dr Qing Li have concluded that forest bathing has numerous physical and mental health benefits. Once you've found a forest or wood close to home, you could make this a regular practice for your wellbeing.

A CLOSER LOOK

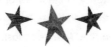

Now you've spent some time in nature, it may be you've noticed a few things that interest you – and it might be time to pay them a little more attention …

> <u>Try this</u>: find something small such as a flower or leaf that you can examine closely. Spend some time looking at your chosen item, observing its colours, shape, texture and smell. You may choose to photograph or draw it. Consider the amazing, exquisite detail it has, as all things have. Ask questions as you observe your object, find out as much as you can about this one small thing just by considering it. If you find your mind drifting away, gently bring it back to your chosen object.

You may find you get curious about certain things as you immerse yourself in nature. Spend time finding out about plants, animals and insects that you love; how they work, what they need to survive and how you can help. The deeper your understanding, you more you will cherish things.

Try this: Stay still, be silent and see what comes to you. You can do this in your own garden as easily as in the park or woods nearby. Observing animals, birds and insects in their natural environment is magical. I sat perfectly still in the woods near my house and watched the squirrels hiding nuts, butterflies chasing each other about; once a fox stopped and sat just a couple of metres away from me. If you enjoy this then check out expert-guided walks – most parks do bat walks and bird walks for those who want to find out more.

Time with animals is relaxing as they don't expect you to be clever or entertaining – you can just be. It still amazes me that we share a planet with such beautiful creatures as cows and deer. You could try walking a friend's dog, horse riding at your local stables, or helping with the animals at a local farm.

A YEAR OF
NATURAL WONDERS

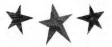

Go in search of wonder: Try a year of seeking out the best that nature has to offer.

Spring

1. Get up and out, and listen to the dawn chorus – the best music ever.
2. Find your nearest bluebell wood and go for a stroll.
3. Visit a pond in the early evening and hear the frogs croaking.

Summer

1. Build a den – noting what you hear, smell and see as you build.
2. Climb a tree – what can you see and hear from up there?
3. Make a rope swing over a stream – enjoy the sun on your skin and the wind in your hair.

Autumn

1. Visit your nearest deer park and see/hear the stags battling, plus enjoy the many colours of the leaves.

2. Look for flocks of jackdaws, rooks and carrion crows flying to woodland roosts in the evenings. At the coast you might see migratory geese arriving from the Arctic.

3. Take an early morning walk and look out for spider webs outlined in dew on hedgerows, branches, house windows and car wing mirrors.

Winter

1. Look out for starling murmurations in the early evening – they tend to happen in places that provide shelter, like woodlands, cliffs, tall buildings and industrial structures.

2. Look out for animal and bird tracks – easy to see in snow and damp soft ground.

3. Go for an evening walk – listen out for woodpeckers drumming and tawny owls hooting and look out for snowdrops.

Lastly, for anytime

Set your alarm and watch the sun rise, or take your time to watch it set. It never fails to impress, especially at the coast or from a hilltop.

CHAPTER 3

CURIOUSER AND CURIOUSER

*Y*ou know when kids keep asking 'but why?', each question leading to another? You might remember being like that yourself, or perhaps you have spent time with a child who is at that stage. This chapter is about (re)discovering that childlike spirit of natural curiosity. All innovation, exploration and discovery begins with somebody, somewhere, asking a question. Curiosity can lead you to some fascinating places and allow you to see the world in a whole new light, with wonder, enthusiasm and delight. Let's begin ...

Your mission

To revisit childhood curiosities and interests. To experience the positive benefits of learning. To share what you've learned with others, and pass on the wonders of knowledge and discovery. To allow yourself to see things you take for granted in a new light. To see where your curiosity takes you ...

ASKING QUESTIONS

Dr Dominic Galliano is a physicist and the director of outreach and public engagement for the South East Physics Network. He is passionate about encouraging all kinds of people to engage with physics, and his definition of what it is to be a scientist chimes with my thoughts about the importance of nurturing your own curiosity and allowing yourself to experience awe and wonder. He told me, 'The first step to becoming a scientist is by asking the question: how does that work?'

My impression from my own work with children is that they are less afraid than adults of being thought 'stupid' or 'silly' for asking questions. Dr Galliano said that many of his colleagues tell him they get the best questions from children – and that these allow more interesting answers, that children are generally less afraid to ask the 'big' questions, like why are we here? What is life? What is the universe?

So I asked Dr Galliano, what happens to us grown-ups? Did we somehow get discouraged from asking questions? Or get too busy? He suggested that the reason this changes is our adult awareness of the existence and certainty of death, and not knowing what happens to us afterwards, and that this fear of mortality gets in the way of us asking big questions. But as we know death is a certainty, we might as well live as well and as fully as we are able, which could include seeking answers and gaining knowledge ...

So let's start by going back to the curiosity of childhood, and see where that leads ...

Alice asked the Cheshire Cat, who was sitting in a tree, 'What road do I take?' The cat asked, 'Where do you want to go?' 'I don't know,' Alice answered. 'Then,' said the cat, 'it really doesn't matter, does it?'

FROM *ALICE'S ADVENTURES IN WONDERLAND* BY LEWIS CARROLL,

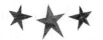

<u>The Big 7</u>: Researchers have identified some questions commonly asked by kids that many adults still don't know the answers to. See how you get on answering these.

1. How is electricity made?
2. Why is the sky blue?
3. How do birds fly?
4. Where does the wind come from?
5. Why do we have dreams?
6. What is time?
7. Where does water come from?

<u>Pass it on</u>: If you found that there was one or more of these you didn't know the answer to – get researching. Once you've got your answers, ask someone else the same question(s) and tell them what you've discovered if they don't know. Think about how you could talk about this explanation to make it interesting to someone else, easy to understand, and get ready to infect someone else with curiosity. An important part of the challenge is to make your answer fascinating for the listener – if you get an 'oh wow' you will have successfully passed on a small piece of wonder.

I am going to find out (or find out more) about …

I am going to share what I discovered with …

It's widely acknowledged that the more you find out about something the greater your appreciation of it. Exploring your curiosities could change your life or career, but it could also simply provide you with an interest that you love. When you allow yourself to be absorbed by curiosity, stress and worries recede.

<u>My questions</u>: I hope those examples reminded you of your own unanswered childhood questions. If they did, then great – you are well on your way to fanning the flames of your curiosity. Note them down and make a start on answering one of them.

The question I asked that never got answered is …

I bet you'll discover that finding answers, especially to long-held questions, is immensely satisfying …

AREAS OF INTEREST

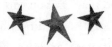

By now you've found out a little about what you do and don't know, and reminded yourself of any unanswered questions you may have had as a child. Before we go further, let's find out some of your interests and passions ...

Interview yourself: Take your time to answer the following questions; the purpose of them is to remind you of broad subjects and areas that you may like to pursue. Answer in as much detail as possible – each of the questions may have several answers.

1. If you could go back to school, what subject would you pay more attention to?
2. If you could choose a different job or occupation (never mind qualifications or other practicalities), what would that be?
3. If you could be a world expert in something, what would that be?

If you wish you'd worked harder in chemistry class, would love to have been a zoo keeper, or would like to be an expert astronomer, the good news is, you can still learn about and develop skills in all of those things, and enrich your life. Choose from one of your answers, and make a start on exploring the subject.

Where to go: Obviously you have the incredible resource of the internet at your disposal, but there are lots of other fun ways of finding stuff out:

- Visit your local public library – ask the librarians for help or just browse.
- Choose one of our incredible (mostly free) national and local museums – check out what special exhibitions they have on. Join their mailing lists.
- Attend a lecture or talk on a subject that interests you. Find out if an author of a book on your subject is doing a talk somewhere.
- Try a short/weekend course in your subject of interest, or a free online course.
- Seek out your local astronomy/history/special interest groups. Chances are they'll be doing loads of events and will be very keen to get new members and ideas. It's a very easy first step to expand your knowledge and a great way of meeting new, like-minded people.

- Subscribe to a magazine for a subject you are curious about, for example an astronomy magazine for news about meteor showers and eclipses. Spend a leisurely hour browsing through the magazine and see what you find interesting.
- Check out the public engagement events on your local University website – there will be free public lectures, festivals and other activities.

Ask yourself:
What do I want to explore ...

Take action:
What I'll do in the next 24 hours (e.g. watch a documentary about the subject) ...

What I am going to do in the next week (e.g. visit a relevant museum or exhibition) ...

What I am going to do in the next month (e.g. attend some talks/start some classes/join an organisation) ...

See where this leads you. It may be that after a month you've found out all you need to know, and are happy to move on to something else, or you may find yourself at the beginning of a longer, possibly life-changing journey.

For the star-gazers out there, check out Galaxy Zoo — it's a crowdsourced astronomy project that invites people to assist in the classification of galaxies; a great example of citizen science (www.zooniverse.org).

<u>A curious year</u>: On the first day of each month for one whole year identify one question you have always wanted the answer to. By the end of the month you must have found the answer. Use this exercise to train your mind to be endlessly curious. Keep a curiosity calendar and see what you learn.

Month	Question	Answer
January		
February		
March		
April		
May		
June		
July		
August		
September		
October		
November		
December		

CLOSER TO HOME

So you've explored what you were curious about as a kid, and hopefully revisited some of those things. You might even have even experienced looking at the stars through a telescope or had your mind blown by a lecture about quantum physics!

However, wonder can also be the feeling of amazement caused by seeing something familiar in a new way, and seeing it as a beautiful or remarkable thing. Curiosity allows you to see that nothing is ordinary. So let's re-examine the everyday things close to home which you take for granted.

As Dr Galliano said: 'Things become even more incredible and impressive when you know what is going on and how they work.'

Every Day Wonders

Choose five things in your home, which you use but don't know how they work. This could be your alarm clock, your laptop, the washing machine or doorbell – it must be something ordinary that you see and/or use every day. Then ask yourself: how does that work?

Prepare the answer like a mini-talk or lecture that you could present to another member of your household or to a friend.

<u>Ask yourself</u>: How did you feel when you were finding out? Did it change the way you feel about the item? How do you feel now you have gained more knowledge? There is no right or wrong answer to these questions, but if the experience of discovery was a positive one you may wish to continue and find out about other things around you.

<u>Everyone's an expert</u>: Expand this exercise to include those you live with: everyone may chose one thing in the house that they are going to find out more about, and each person has one week to do so. Arrange to get together at the end of the week and take it in turns to share your new knowledge with each other.

<u>A curious tea party</u>: As well as bringing food to share, each guest's contribution is that they bring one weird or wonderful fact, and one question they would love to know the answer to. Everyone leaves having learnt something (and having had delicious grub, of course). If there are any unanswered questions, one guest agrees to find the answer ready for next time you have your party. Have fun sending out your invitation – who would be the five most interesting people to invite?

Curiosity is, in great and
generous minds, the first
passion and the last.

WILLIAM SAMUEL JOHNSON

CHAPTER 4

PRACTICAL MAGIC

*I*f you were lucky, when you were a child, your belief in magic was encouraged. Your stories were filled with wizards, unicorns and other magical creatures. As an adult you might still enjoy those kinds of stories but you probably don't 'believe' in the same way.

When you see someone make a coin disappear in front of your very eyes, you understand that the trick isn't 'real', yet I bet you still experience the thrill of the spectacle and enjoy being lifted out of the ordinary and entertained. In fact, once you realise that to make the trick work requires hundreds of hours of painstaking practice, it can be even more amazing! You know it's a trick, you might even know how it was done, but it is still awe-inspiring.

Research has revealed that in order to survive, humans need to make sense of the world. When you can't explain things logically (how did that rabbit appear from the hat, when I saw with my own eyes that the hat was empty before?) but you know you're safe (in a theatre), you experience the pleasure of awe and wonder. This can lift your mood and relieve stress.

This chapter is an invitation to spread some wonder by trying out your own magic tricks on friends and strangers, and have a great time while doing so. Don't worry – you won't have to practise sleight of hand for months in your bedroom! To explore this idea I chatted with my magician friends Kane Sinclair-Sojka and Philipp Oberlohr – they both spoke about the fun and joy to be had from performing magic; I hope you will experience this too. Our conversations inspired the following exercises, all tried and tested by me. I believe they are suitable for kids or adults, and encourage you to try them with both.

Your mission:

Using creative and practical exercises, make some magic of your own. Discover the joy of spreading wonder, lifting yourself and others out of the ordinary and by doing so allowing magic back into your life.

BECOMING A MAGICIAN
– FIRST THINGS FIRST

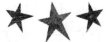

For fun, I invite you to create your own magical name. You may want to use it to increase the mystery of your tricks, for example when signing things or leaving messages etc.

<u>How to create your magical name</u>: Choose a positive adjective followed by your favourite teacher's name (e.g. The Magnificent Ms Hibdidge).

My magic name is: _____

Also, if you have a dramatic flair, maybe you'd like a special outfit?

Your look could be a billowing velvet cape, a sharp suit or a glittery jumpsuit. You decide.

My outfit/look is: _____

Of course, feel free to use your own, perfectly good name, and to wear your own, perfectly interesting clothes if you'd prefer. Not all magicians wear sequins, after all.

Three Rules for the Magician – refer to these when in doubt:

1. Use the element of surprise.

2. Rehearse/plan your trick before you carry it out.

3. Never knowingly repeat the same trick to the same audience twice.

The moment you doubt whether
you can fly, you cease for ever
to be able to do it.

FROM *PETER PAN* BY J.M. BARRIE,

MAGICAL GIFTS

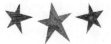

Now you know the basics, and you might even have a name and an outfit, so you're ready to try some tricks. Start by trying some of these gift ideas on friends, but don't feel you have to wait for a special occasion or a birthday. You'll see as you try them out how simple it is to transform someone's day with the magic of kindness and generosity.

I have come to understand
that real magic is just
human kindness.

KANE SINCLAIR-SOJKA, MAGICIAN

1. Decorate the path to someone's home with flowers, candles, beautiful objects, or drawings.
2. If you know someone who travels the same journey every day, leave messages on station platforms, lampposts, walls and fences for them to see en route.
3. Decorate someone's window so that when they open their curtains they'll have a surprise! You could paint a picture, create a collage of images or photographs, or write something for them.
4. Create a treasure hunt at home by leaving clues leading to a prize.
5. Send an anonymous invitation to a friend, telling them to be at a designated rendezvous point at a certain date/time. Surprise them with a night/day out, being as daring as time and budget allow.
6. Created and post a video online for someone – it could be you singing 'Happy Birthday', telling them a story, or some footage of their favourite place or view. Give them the link to the film.
7. Give someone a dice and a list of treats they could have depending on which number they roll!

Magic is a way of engineering surprise. Research has revealed that surprise is good for us, by working on the dopamine system in our brains; it helps us to focus our attention and inspires us to be curious, and to see the world and our situation differently.

Kindness is a sort of magic,
because of the transformations
that kindness can achieve.

PHILIPP OBERLOHR, ILLUSIONIST

TRICKS AS TREATS

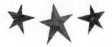

Lift someone out of their ordinary day by surprising them with a bit of 'magic'!

<u>Try these</u>:
- Sneak a small gift into someone's bag, car, gym kit or lunch box.
- Fill someone's favourite cup with some treats.
- Transform a drawer or cupboard in your home. Empty the usual things out – then get decorating with drawings, images or wrapping paper. You could fill it with cakes, homemade gifts or messages. As an example: my friend Annie hung a mirror ball in her understairs cupboard and transformed it into 'disco land' complete with silver curtains and other decorations as a surprise for her sister's birthday.

<u>Away with the faeries</u>: In the spirit of the unpredictable, anarchic, wild-eyed version of faeries you find in old folk tales, here is a good trick for a friend who needs cheering up.

Leave faerie footprints on someone's windowsill – all you need is glitter* and some doll shoes. Put the glitter on the shoes and tread a path from your friend's window leading to a note, like this:

Dear Emma, it has come to our attention that you are not feeling so good and we're sorry to hear that. Remember that you have friends and are loved. Best wishes, the (insert place here) **faeries.**

Then roll up the note and tie it with string.
*Some glitter is made rom tiny pieces of plastic, which is not good for the environment. You can however get eco-friendly glitter now (see the back of the book for suggestions) or you could use water-soluble paint instead.

HOW TO BECOME
A FAIRY GODPARENT

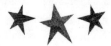

Offer to be a wise and kindly protector for someone as their very own Fairy Godparent – a kind of magical mentor.

Try this: First, identify someone who you think would like this and make the offer. Devise a contract for them, with an outline of what you are offering, e.g.:

I offer you the following:
Wise and sensible advice at any time.
Someone to call at 2am when you absolutely have to.
Somewhere to stay when you need to.
Encouragement and flattery ...

If they accept the offer, congratulations. You are now a Fairy Godparent.

A large part of your job is making wishes come true. Sounds a bit … impossible, I know. But wishes are useful in that they reveal what we want – once we know that, we can work out a way of fulfilling them. Our wishes can deliver us to our future.

Try this: offer them three wishes, promising that you will help make them come true as best you can. Get to the bottom of the wishes by asking questions and listening. Here's an example:

I wish I were rich.
Why?
Because then I wouldn't have to work.
Why?
Because I don't like my job.
OK. So let's work out together how to get you into a job that you enjoy.

Now it's over to you to help them work out the next part of their journey. Enjoy your Fairy Godparenting – you could transform someone's life with your help and advice.

The most important thing in life is
to stop saying 'I wish' and start saying
'I will'. Consider nothing impossible,
then treat possibilities as probabilities.

CHARLES DICKENS

I hope by now you've enjoyed yourself trying out some
'magic' on friends and loved ones. Now I dare you to go out
into the wide world and try some tricks out there, starting
with the power of magic words …

ALL WORDS ARE
MAGIC WORDS

Words can transform someone's unhappiness into joy, when chosen carefully. Use yours to spread some wonder with these exercises.

Try this: Leave notes on park benches, at bus stops, under pillows, etc. Consider what to write in relation to the kind of response you hope for – do you want to encourage or inspire people? Or make them laugh? Write 'read me' on the envelope for extra mystery. Other fun places to leave notes are:

- Inside library books
- In shops
- On tables or chairs in cafés
- On train, bus, plane and tram seats
- On cinema or theatre seats
- At the dentist's or doctor's
- Inside the pockets of coats in charity shops
- On community noticeboards

<u>Magic letters</u>: We mostly just get pizza adverts and bills through the post these days. This is what makes letter writing and receiving so special.

Try this:
- Write to a friend from a 'secret admirer' – making sure the recipient is the kind of person who'd enjoy the mystery!
- Write interesting letters to strangers, leaving them where they're most likely to be found.
- Write a letter to someone you admire and tell them the reasons you do.

STREET MAGIC

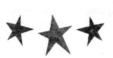

Next, try these exercises and transform the everyday environment into a wonderland. They're fun to do with friends – you can create some dramatic visual spectacles even quicker with a few people helping out!

Doll power: Get some old dolls (any kind) and make them some placards using lolly sticks and blank postcards. Decide what kind of message you'll write on the placards – what would you like them to say? Attach the placards to the dolls' hands with elastic bands, then the dolls to railings, fences, trees etc. with cable ties or string.

Transformations: Make a public place beautiful by decorating or transforming it – for example, I've created cafés in phone boxes, and covered park benches in flowers and sequins, or tied luggage labels with messages to trees and bushes. Make sure you choose a place that gets lots of passers-by for maximum impact.

I hope you enjoyed getting creative and trying out some magic. Next we will be moving on to look at the wonder of the arts ...

CHAPTER 5

WE ARE ALL ARTISTS

*L*ike a lot of kids, I loved drawing and making up stories. I still remember writing a story about a vegetarian dinosaur, and spending hours painting a picture of a girl who had turned into a tree. It didn't cross my mind to worry about whether or not I was 'good' at any of these things, I just loved doing them, was proud of being able to share the results, and often amazed at what I had achieved.

I've been fortunate as an adult to be able to make my living in various creative ways, and have loved and appreciated my jobs, but I still get the most pleasure out of putting aside any goals or ambition to get lost in being creative, in the moment.

This chapter is an invitation to enjoying the arts for their own sake and for their therapeutic benefits.

Your mission:

To explore your creativity in many different ways. To experience how being creative can inspire and enrich your life, and how you can inspire others by sharing your creativity.

I'm a fan of all forms of creativity, from cake-decorating to sculpture, poetry to pottery and everything in between. Psychologists have found that when you get totally immersed in something creative, you find yourself in a meditative-like state of 'flow', which focuses you and pushes aside all your worries for a while. Creativity increases the 'feelgood' neurotransmitter dopamine, which explains why art feels good. The arts have also been found to help you find solutions and invent, they inspire, motivate, and help you express difficult memories or complicated emotions. It helps you see the world in a new light and experience ordinary things in an extraordinary way.

GET INSPIRED

Whether you are already a professional artist, or someone who would never think of themselves as creative, I'd like you to begin by experiencing as many kinds of art as possible.

<u>Your big art adventure</u>: Ask a few people to name their favourite piece of music, poem, song, painting, statue, film, novel etc. Collect ideas from as wide a range of people as possible. Variety will make it more interesting – a twelve-year-old may well have a very different list to a fifty-year-old. Create a record of what they chose:

Name	Recommends	Tick (when checked it out)

A study by neurobiologists revealed that experiencing art we enjoy produces pleasure similar to falling in love. All the arts can elevate us out of the ordinary into a state of heightened perception, a perpetual state of wonder, whereby even a bus journey on a rainy evening can be transformed if you are listening to a beautiful piece of music.

Keep an inspiration journal: keep images or ideas in a scrapbook or online – Pinterest and Instagram are fantastic platforms for collecting ideas. Take note when something makes you think 'I could do/would like to do that', but also allow yourself to simply enjoy!

Just in case you're thinking, 'but I don't have time to be creative!' I promise that you should be able to fit the following exercises into a regular day. You may amaze yourself with what you can do.

Monday: make a one-minute film on your smartphone of something you find beautiful.

Tuesday: take ten photos which tell the story in pictures of where you live.

Wednesday: write a portrait of someone you love on one side of A4 lined paper.

Thursday: draw a picture of one item in your home which you see every day.

Friday: find a piece of music which you think would work as the theme song to your day today.

Saturday: copy out the lyrics of your favourite song, and speak them aloud as a poem.

Sunday: transform a room in you home using just what is available – give yourself an hour to do so.

Notice which of those you most enjoyed, which you found easy or more challenging, if there were any you'd like to try again and if you were surprised by anything.

ART AT HOME

You don't need special equipment or a workshop to begin your own creative projects — you can start with what you already have, in your own home. I talked with visual artist Stephen Wright about this, and the importance of allowing yourself to be creative. He told me about outsider art, which is made by people from all walks of life who created because they felt they had to, often inspired by dreams and visions, using materials that others might throw away. Stephen told me he admired the 'childlike wonder' of this art. He created his own incredibly beautiful environment, 'The House of Dreams', in London (visit www.stephenwrightartist.com to find out more). Stephen's home is both a gallery and museum, and demonstrates that you can make art anywhere, out of anything. Stephen said: 'it's important to allow yourself to play, to enjoy creativity for its own sake, for the pleasure of it ... and to make yourself time in a busy world. You don't need permission from anyone else to be creative, you just need courage.'

Why not use your home as your canvas as Stephen has?

For art at home try these:

- Create a scrapbook with photographs and memorabilia, choosing to tell the story of your year, or of a special time, or your family history.
- Paint a mural on a wall, with images or quotes that will inspire you.
- Sew a patchwork quilt out of clothes you no longer wear.
- Create a collage of images that express how you are feeling or tell a story. Use old magazines, photographs or drawings.

WONDER TALES

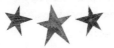

We've learned from anthropologists that storytelling is a part of being human. We tell stories to share our understanding of the world with each other. Scientists have found that when we are listening to a story, rather than simply facts or figures, our brains are much more engaged. This is why stories can inspire us, affect our emotions and change our ideas about things. The following exercises are inspired by professional storyteller Vanessa Woolf, with whom I've had the pleasure of working many times. Vanessa tells her magical stories to adults and children in surprising and wonderful places and is extremely passionate about the power of oral storytelling.

> <u>My favourite</u>: Pick a story you've heard that you enjoyed, one that resonates with you. Write down the key points to help you remember, then re-tell it your own way to a friend, someone who will be receptive and supportive. Keep it short.
>
> <u>Are you sitting comfortably?</u>: Offer to read stories to children from books, re-tell a story you love, or one you've created. Try

your library, a school, children's hospital or playgroup nearby. Try the stories out on the children in your life and see what works best.

<u>Fireside</u>: Start a story circle. Invite a group of friends round and tell a five-minute story each. Make it a monthly meet-up, in a community space, someone's home, or best of all, outside around a fire.

Stories are a wonderful way for us to reconnect with magic and wonder. They are as essential for us as sunlight.

VANESSA WOOLF

If you prefer to write, get yourself a notebook and keep it with you always. Try the following ways of sparking your storytelling creativity:

Overheard: Note any exchanges of conversation that intrigue you. You might want to use one of these conversations as the beginning of a story, script or poem.

The writing's on the wall: Record all the writing you see in public – signs like 'danger do not enter' or graffiti like 'Mary loves Sally'. Choose one and use it as a starting point for a creative writing exercise. (The story of where Mary met Sally, for example.)

Recycling: Cut up a couple of damaged books into sentences you like. Choose ten at random, and then out of those words create a poem/song that makes sense to you. You may want to throw in a few extra words to make your poem/song flow better. Give it a title.

THE TWO OF US

It's great fun, and beneficial for your relationship, to create with someone. Being inspired and encouraged by a supportive partner may take you even further with your ideas ... art history is populated by incredible partnerships inspiring each other. So pair up and get started ...

- Challenge your partner to respond creatively to a specific theme, e.g. summer. They then challenge you in turn with a different theme. Each of you may respond in any way you like, so long as it fits the given theme (parameters can be very helpful to the creative process, in that they give you a starting point. How far you travel is up to you!). Decide on a deadline between you – then go for it!

- Decide on a joint theme that you would both like to work on. Work separately, then come together at an agreed time and see what you've each come up with. You don't have to be working in the same medium – imagine how interesting it could be if a musician and a knitter both created something on the theme of 'stormy weather'!

- Play creative tag – you create something, and then present it to your partner. They then use that as inspiration, respond creatively, then present it back, and repeat for as long as you both like. For example: Dave shows me his painting of a butterfly – I respond by writing a story about the rainforest, he draws a picture of a monkey, I write a story about a chimp in a circus … etc. See where it leads you both.

If you've enjoyed working in a pair, and are intrigued by the possibilities of creating with others, try these ideas and experience the joy of group creativity.

FIND YOUR TRIBE

Some art forms lend themselves more easily to collaboration, and some need different people with different skills to make them happen, The joy of the shared experience, and the depth of friendships once you've had that shared experience of creating something together, is incredible. Join an existing group, or create your own.

D.I.Y.: Start something creative with a small group of like-minded friends – propose a regular meet and the members of the group who are able could take it in turn to host. You could offer to teach and exchange skills with each other.

If you've yet to find people with shared interests, find an existing group by looking online or at community noticeboards to see what is going on in your area.

<u>All the world's a stage</u>: Check out your local 'am dram' group – most hold regular auditions. There are plenty of opportunities for acting, dancing and singing, plus all the backstage jobs. If carpentry, costumes, prop making, directing, composing or choreography are your thing, there will be a place for you there. Offer your existing skills, or say you'd like to learn! Start by seeing a production so you're familiar with their work.

<u>Sing</u>: check out your local community choirs – they usually sing all kinds of music and welcome all ages. Or invite a group of friends around to sing – print off lyric sheets and get some backing tracks to some well-known classics. If you love playing an instrument you could find a community orchestra or local bands.

I hope this chapter has provided you with a provocation to be creative, and that it has inspired your own ideas. Being creative can make you fully alive to the wonder of human existence. Remember, art is whatever we say it is. Be freed by that knowledge.

One ought, every day at least, to
hear a little song, read a good poem,
see a fine picture, and, if it were
possible, to speak a few
reasonable words.

JOHANN WOLFGANG VON GOETHE

CHAPTER 6

THE ROAD LESS TRAVELLED

We live on a planet with seven different continents, and 195 countries. We share it with more than 7 billion people, who speak thousands of languages. We've so far discovered over 8.7 million other species here too. Every day every living creature on earth has their own set of unique experiences of which we are unaware. What a wonderful world it is.

In spite of this, for the most part, we stick to what we know. We wonder why we feel a little stale and unstimulated at times.

You probably have a routine too. You may go to bed and get up around the same time most days, go the same route to work or college, eat the same sort of food, and do similar activities in your spare time. There's good reason for this – it's easier to organise life that way, plus the way society is structured dictates at least some of those routines, they work and are comfortable, so why change them?

However, wonder rarely resides in routine. You need to tip things upside down and shake them a little, like a snow globe, and then you see the magic. If you feel bored or restless, and that your routine is no longer a comfort but a chore, or even if you like things as they are but are prepared to disrupt them a little, you might change your life. How much is up to you. Let's begin ...

Your mission:

To disrupt your life in order to see things from a fresh perspective. To allow yourself to wonder what might happen if you dare to follow your dreams, and to explore ways of beginning to do so.

The real voyage of discovery
consists not in seeking
new landscapes but in
having new eyes.

MARCEL PROUST

GENTLE DISRUPTIONS

The following exercises are to allow you to see your life, yourself and the world from a different angle. You might simply have fun, or discover things you'd like to incorporate into your life. Have a look through first and do any preparation you might need for your 'week of wonders'.

Start off by trying one of these each day:

Monday: try the most interesting, beautiful or unusual way to make your regular, everyday journey. Take a different train, cycle if you usually drive, or leave earlier and walk, etc. Observe as much as possible on the way, such as birds, buildings, the sky, and your fellow travellers.

Tuesday: carry out one act of kindness for a stranger today. You'll have to be present in the moment so that you don't miss the opportunity to do so when it arises. It doesn't have to be a grand or extravagant thing – it can be small.

Wednesday: phone a friend, someone you wish you kept in closer touch with. Set aside time to chat. If you can't speak, write.

Thursday: visit somewhere in your neighbourhood that you have never been before – a park, wildlife reserve, interesting street, etc. Be a tourist at home.

Friday: have a chat with a total stranger – good openings are talking about the weather or telling them you like something they are wearing.

Decide for yourself if any of the above are 'keepers' – if they were beneficial or fun you could make them part of your daily life. Whenever you begin to get bored or restless, try them again. The next exercises will take a little more preparation and time:

Saturday: partner up with a friend and take it in turns to devise a 'day of wonders' for each other, packed with as many surprises as possible.

Sunday: you can do this alone or with a partner. Write ten things that you'd love to do; the rules are that they have to be doable in one day and they have to be ambitious, but not impossible (so that rules out 'become invisible', for example!) Put the ideas into a hat, pick one at random and do it. You might want to choose the day before in case you need to prepare. Continue for as long as you wish, topping up with new ideas as they come. As you become more confident, you may want to make the ideas even more daring and ambitious.

I DARE YOU

If you're feeling daring and up for an adventure, try these. The first exercise is one I've done every time I've been travelling as well as at home. As a result I once spent a day having a milkshake with a blues musician, visiting a haunted pub, and delivering a bar of chocolate to a girl I'd never met before who worked in a coffee shop.

<u>Wild days</u>: Find somewhere lively and full of people, close to home. Choose a friendly-looking stranger and ask them to recommend somewhere for you to go. Explain that you only have one day, but you'd like an adventure. Once you get the recommendation, go, enjoy that destination, and repeat. That's it. Before you begin, make sure someone knows you're doing it and agree to check in with them at a specified time, just to be safe. Decide on your budget for the day, pack and dress for any eventuality (layers, snacks, and sensible footwear).

Here's something I do every year to shake things up ...

When you try new things, you are placing yourself into situations where you are forced to think, which stimulates creativity. You'll find trying out new things helps you see everything in a new light. You are giving yourself the opportunity to discover, grow and be stimulated, and to experience wonder.

SWEET DREAMS

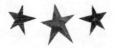

I hope that by now you've experienced how even small changes are good for you and can be mind-expanding.

How about the big changes you might need to make if you want to live the life of your dreams? I think it's worth checking that our long-held dreams can still serve us well before we consider how to pursue them.

For example, let's say your dream is to be a pop star. Even amazing singers who want to be pop stars have no guarantee of making a living from it. But if you understood that the reason behind you wanting to be a pop star was that you wanted a more exciting life, you could then consider other, possibly easier choices that might serve that purpose too.

So what is *your* dream? Consider what's at the heart of it and then you can explore the many paths that might get you where you'd like to be.

My dream is: _____
_____
_____
_____

Because I want: _____

Some other ways I could get what I want:
_____
_____
_____
_____

I think you should let yourself have more dreams, and new ones, and let go of those that no longer serve you well. I hope that the exercise demonstrated that there are many paths to a desired destination (and I'd say choose the easiest!).

Dreams provide us with focus and purpose and can also help us get through difficult times, so use yours to motivate you.

Louise Dumayne left her life in London and an acting career behind her to realise her childhood dream of living in the wilderness. (You can read about Louise's adventures here: www.yukonbushlife.com.)

If you really want to change things but your nerves are failing you, here are some top tips I learned from Louise:

<u>Consider the worst-case scenario</u>: if you pursued your dream to the fullest, what is the worst that could happen? (Ruling out death, which could happen to anyone, anytime, and therefore doesn't count.) Ask yourself if you could live with it, and if the answer is yes, go for it.

<u>Rehearse</u>: soldiers rehearse for battle, and actors rehearse for their big opening, because 'practice makes perfect'. If you want to swim the Channel, make a start by rehearsing lengths in the pool.

<u>Take small steps</u>: do what is comfortable – too big a leap can feel scary; even making a small change is moving you in the right direction. If you feel you have to make a huge leap it can put you off doing anything.

<u>Take your time</u>: create and carve out time to consider what you want and need. Go at your own pace.

We should give ourselves permission to dream, and allow ourselves the things that will make us happy. This isn't selfish, it is about living our lives to the fullest we can.

LOUISE DUMAYNE

CHAPTER 7

POSITIVE THINKING

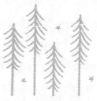

I believe that thinking negatively can cut us off from experiencing life fully, locking us into fear and sadness. The joy of experiencing wonder is much better served by thinking positively. I talked about the benefits of positive thinking with Dr Ruth Wareham, a philosopher of education at Warwick University. She told me: 'There's a Greek word *eudaimonia*, it's most commonly translated as happiness, but a more accurate translation has been proposed which is "human flourishing or living well".' I kept this word and our conversation in mind when considering the value of positive thinking. Thinking positively doesn't mean living in denial or refusing to acknowledge negative events or feelings, nor does it mean being happy all of the time. It's a way of being which improves your strength and resilience and allows you to live a 'flourishing life'. Life has obstacles, challenges, difficulties, pain, some things we would just rather have not happened. It also contains rewards, opportunities, unexpected joy, nice surprises, and great beauty. It is rich and varied, and that is every human being's experience.

Our emotions are complex. Anger can be motivating, sadness can help us heal. However, I believe that working through whatever comes your way to a positive way of thinking about things is empowering and informative. It can be as simple as 'this is painful, but it won't last'. Thinking positively as often as you are able gives you strength and frees you to appreciate the wonder around you every day in every moment.

This chapter is about aiming to see the positive side of everything and to work towards seeking solutions to problems whenever possible.

Your mission:

To learn to think positively about yourself, your community and the wider world, to develop strategies for combating negative news, and to appreciate that the world is still a wonderful place by doing so.

POSITIVELY YOU

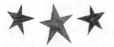

Practise positive thinking towards yourself. If you find negative self-talk popping up, gently replace it with positive affirmations, remind yourself of your skills, talents and achievements. Things you haven't yet achieved are opportunities, not things to punish yourself with. Ask yourself what you might like to improve upon, learn about, and do, in order to enrich your life and increase the possibility of experiencing wonder – what would inspire you?

<u>Answer these</u>:

Something I do that I would like to get better at is …

Something I would love to learn is …

A new experience I would love to have is …

_____

_____

_____

<u>Little acorns</u>: make a start on each of these. Start small, for example planting a window box or going for a swim once a week. This small achievement will pay dividends – even a small achievement or success causes your brain to release dopamine, which is what that little rush of pleasure is, and this keeps you motivated.

Write your ideas here:

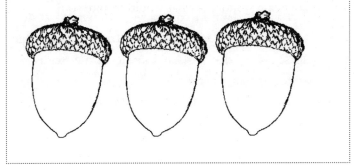

Now is the time to understand more,
so that we may fear less.

MARIE CURIE

It may feel a little daunting or scary – we humans do tend to crave the familiar. Don't be afraid to go slowly. Once you've made a start, decide what your next little step is, and continue, for as long as you wish.

FEAR AND CURIOSITY

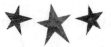

You may have found when you tried the 'little acorn' exercises that you experienced a twinge of fear. Some fears are useful, of course, and keep you out of harm's way, e.g. 'I'm scared of getting cancer, so I stopped smoking.' Others are illogical – 'I'm afraid that no one will employ me as a gardener so I won't do the horticulture course.'

Sort your useful fears (keeping you out of *real* harm's way) from your not-so-useful fears (stopping you from doing things by imagining problems that don't exist yet).

Curiosity is the best way to combat fear. What if you give up your job and go travelling? What if you say yes to the invitation? What happens then?

It is not death that a man
should fear, but he should
fear never beginning to live.

MARCUS AURELIUS

<u>Try exploring your fears:</u> What are you afraid of? Does fear stop you doing things that might be good for you or fun? Try filling this in for each of the things you are most afraid of.

I'm afraid of …

_____

_____

This is stopping me …

_____

_____

This is a good thing because …

_____

_____

This is a bad thing because …

_____

_____

Then ask yourself: does the good outweigh the bad? Is this fear improving your life? Or would your life be better without it? Is it worth trying the thing you're afraid of? What if …

_____

_____

_____

Here are some simple exercises to combat fears and to shake you out of your 'comfort zone' into the 'wonder zone'.

The wonder of no: If you find you often say YES to things you don't want to do, then try saying no and using the time to do something you *really* would like to instead. Just try one 'no' in place of your usual 'yes' in the next month.

The wonder of yes: Try saying yes to an invitation you would normally decline – you could discover a new hobby, make new friends, or simply have a great time. Saying yes requires turning up and engaging in the activity too, giving yourself the chance to enjoy it. Try one 'yes' in the next month.

Most research concludes that thinking positively may help you better cope with stress, which reduces its harmful effects on your body and mind. Having a positive outlook reduces your risk of cardiovascular diseases, and optimistic people tend to exercise more, eat healthier food and smoke and drink less. Thinking positively has the potential to give you a longer and happier life.

A POSITIVE WORLD

Whatever positive feelings you have about yourself and your life will be hugely increased if you engage positively with the big wide world out there.

Let's start with your little patch of it. We can sometimes feel negatively about where we live (in a 'the grass is always greener' way) but wonders surround us everywhere, in nature, buildings and people. Find yours.

<u>My little patch of wonder</u>:

Three amazing things about my community/local area are:

....

....

....

Three wonderful things about my home town/country are:

....

....

....

Three positive facts about people in my community are:

....

....

....

Remind yourself of these when and if you feel downhearted or discouraged – remember how fortunate you are. Now let's consider the wider world …

<u>News of the world</u>: We are bombarded with negative news. A redressing of the balance is called for; it doesn't require a denial of reality or of the facts, but it does require seeking possible solutions and a call to positive action, which is empowering and hopeful. Try these and note how by doing them you feel differently.

- Many of us are turning away from the news because we can't take the negativity. There is a healthy antidote to that which you can be part of – lots of individuals and organisations are committed to reporting only positive news, solutions-driven journalism, hope-filled stories about people doing good, and informed and reasonable debate. Seek them out.

- Be a positive newshound by seeking out one positive story a week and then share it. Focus on what *you're* interested in: scientific innovations, stories from the natural world or humans being wonderful.
- If a piece of news is filling you with despair then seek out the hope or possible solutions. Share what you find.

The bright side: It's possible to train yourself into a more positive way of thinking by committing to looking on the bright side. Try these:

- Seek out stories about people doing amazing, positive things. If you feel inspired, find out how they achieved them and how it would be possible for you to the same. Surround yourself with people who find the positive in things too.
- Find the positive in every circumstance, everything that happens and in every experience. Think of it as a workout for your positivity – creating a magical shield of protection against negativity. There always is some good, somewhere, even though it is difficult to see sometimes.
- List things you don't like in one column. Then create a new column right next to that titled 'on the bright side': write the positive side of each. If you're struggling, get a friend to help. Practise finding the positive.

The bad news is ...	But on the bright side ...

Reasons to be cheerful: it really is a wonderful world, and it is very good to be aware of this.

<u>Here's a challenge</u>: find a different wonder of the world every day for a week. Once you've done that and if you enjoyed it, try doing it for a month. Then a year. I guarantee that you will never run out of wonders, and you will find it is a very positive way of thinking. Here's a few for starters:

1. A café in Scotland has built an eco-village for their homeless employees. They also donate 100 per cent of their proceeds to charity and have provided over 100,000 items of free food to the homeless in the last twelve months.

2. Trees in a forest communicate and share resources through an underground network built by soil fungi. 'Mother' trees support young seedlings by sending excess nutrients to them via this network.

3. Elephants experience emotions such as loss, grieving and crying. When the 'Elephant Whisperer' Lawrence Anthony died, a herd of elephants arrived at his house to mourn him.

4. By 1966 the population of blue whales had fallen to 400. That year decisions were made in London to legally protect them from commercial hunting. Now there are around 20,000. In the Natural History Museum in London the skeleton of a blue whale called Hope is on display, as a symbol of our power to have a positive impact on the earth.

Start your own list of Wonders of the World here:

WONDERS WILL
NEVER CEASE

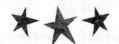

Thank you so much for reading this book. I hope you enjoyed exploring wonder. I hope that many people will allow themselves to do so, and as a result will come to take better care of themselves, each other and the world.

Sometimes all it takes is for us to see or do something differently for everything to change for the better.

Make us aware of the magic, mystery
and wonder of the world … to see
the ordinary as extraordinary,
the familiar as strange, the
mundane as sacred, the
finite as infinite.

NOVALIS

FURTHER READING

ONLINE

For happiness-related features: www.greatergood.berkeley.edu

For citizen science ideas: www.zooniverse.org

For eco-friendly glitter: www.ecoglitterfun.com

For stargazing: www.darkskydiscovery.org.uk

For an inspiring and inclusive art project:
   www.windowwanderland.com

For positive news: https://balance.media and
   www.positive.news

For tree planting etc.: www.treesforcities.org

For inspiring and inclusive arts projects to get involved in, try:
   www.windowwanderland.com or www.funpalaces.co.uk

BOOKS

A New Map of Wonders by Caspar Henderson

Wonders of The Solar System by Professor Brian Cox

Art As Therapy by Alain de Botton and John Armstrong

The Tao of Pooh by Benjamin Hoff

ACKNOWLEDGEMENTS

Many thanks to all these amazing people below who put up with my daft questions, drank tea with me and helped me with the writing of this book.

Dr Bentley Crudgington (@Incidentallyb) , Kate Baily (www. lovesober.com), Lucy Minshall-Pearson (Natural History Museum, London), Dr Dominic Galliano (@PhysicsDom), Kane Sinclair-Sojka (www.youtube.com/user/BlackBoxMagicUK), Philipp Oberlohr (http://philippoberlohr.com/wordpress/), Stephen Wright (www.stephenwrightartist.com), Vanessa Woolf (https:// londondreamtime.com), Louise Dumayne (http://yukonbushlife. com) and Dr Ruth Wareham (Warwick University).

Also huge thanks to the following people who have advised me, made me laugh, employed me and looked after me during this year of wonder.

Ed Cobbold, Flo Schroeder, Kate Jones, Suzanne Keyte, Elizabeth Harper and the rest of the team at the Royal Albert Hall, plus the wonderful Emma Cooper, the staff (and exhibits) of the Natural History Museum; Matt Feerick and Judy Barrington Smuts of www.wetpicnic.com and all my lovely co-conspirators at Crime Scene Live – Graeme Cockburn, Mary Eddowes, Ana Mirtha Sariego, Janine Fletcher, Ross Flight, Chris Montague, Paul Hamilton, Olivia Furber; also Patrick Armstrong, Camilla

Al-Hariri, and the students of Open Stages at King Solomon Academy; Catarina Sousa, Denis Kane, and the participants at Penfold Community Hub, Karen Taylor and Mabel for walks in the woods and words of wisdom; Dan Thompson and Rob Kennedy for marching and making art with me; Kelsey Nagy and Laurie Legocki for looking after me in the US where the idea for this book began to grow as I visited with goats, saw bears and looked out over the Beartooth Mountains; Deptford Folk and Trees for Cities for your great work and for teaching me how to plant a tree; Sophie Austin and Teatro Vivo for inviting me into the Faerie Den; Lucy Nicholls and Antonia Beck for helping me think about how brilliant it is to be alive, Paul Forster and That's What She Said for inviting me to tell stories; Sarah Corbett for support, bubbly and inspiration; Sophie Scott and Dahlia Cuby from *Balance* magazine for kindness and support; Gill Lloyd , Mary Osborn, Chief Dawethi and Pete Staves from Arts Admin for providing me with a home from home, Brookmill Studio and Deptford X for giving me a space to work; Martin Hoenle and Festa Sul Prato for letting me hang out and write, Noera, Helen and Moern from Addis Taste for their delicious vegan Ethiopian food; Amelia Pimlott and Hannah Marshall of Ding Foundation, Jane Corry and the rest of 'Team Moomin' at Norden Farm, Darin Jewell my hard-working agent; Olivia Morris, Leanne Oliver and the amazing, inspiring team at Orion Spring; my sisters Natalie and Kimberley and brothers-in-law Ian and Chris, and my mum Jackie and her partner Graham, for being hilarious; George, Josie, William and Ella for being inspiring and adorable;

Christine 'Wonder' Entwisle, Paschale Straiton, and everyone else who was part of 'Are You Sitting Comfortably?' – look what we started ...

Special thanks to Lola the dog for walking with me every day.

All my friends and neighbours in Deptford.

And last but by no means least, thanks to my lovely Gareth, for reading me Scottish fairy tales all those years ago, and for always having a story to tell me.

This book is dedicated to my friend Chahine Yavroyan, who makes magic happen wherever he is.

ABOUT THE AUTHOR

Bernadette Russell is an author, performer and thaumaturge who lives in Deptford, south-east London, where she writes and creates performances for both adults and children. She has made shows for the Royal Albert Hall, the National Theatre, the Southbank Centre and Birmingham Rep among many others. She's an award-winning kindness campaigner and a columnist for *Balance* magazine. To find out more about Bernadette and her work, visit:

www.bernadetterussell.com – where you can read about all of her solo projects, books, blog and podcasts

www.366daysofkindness.com – where you can read all about the kindness project

www.thewhiterabbit.org.uk – where you can read about the work of her arts organisation

You can find her on Instagram @bernadetterussell or Facebook @bernadetterussellwrites or join her on Twitter @betterussell and share your wonders using #littlewonders.

ALSO BY BERNADETTE RUSSELL

Be inspired by the power of kindness

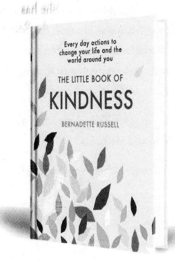